UNDERSTANDING POSTINOR 2

A Comprehensive Guide to Emergency Contraception

CONTENTS

CHAPTER ONE

UNDERSTANDING POSTINOR 2

1.1 What is Postinor 2?

A. Definition and Purpose

Postinor 2 is an emergency contraceptive pill used to prevent pregnancy after unprotected sex or contraceptive failure (e.g., a condom break). It contains the active ingredient levonorgestrel, a synthetic hormone that helps prevent ovulation, fertilization, or implantation of a fertilized egg. It is intended for use as a backup method and not as a regular form of contraception.

1.2 History and Development

Postinor 2 was developed as a more accessible and effective form of emergency contraception. Initially, high-dose combined oral contraceptives were used for emergency contraception, but they often caused significant side effects. In the 1970s, researchers began exploring the use of progestin-only formulations, leading to the development of levonorgestrel-based emergency contraceptives. Postinor 2 was introduced to provide a reliable, easy-to-use option for women needing emergency contraception.

1.3 How Does It Work?

A. Mechanism of Action

Postinor 2 works primarily by preventing or delaying ovulation. If ovulation has already occurred, it may also inhibit fertilization by altering the function of the fallopian tubes. Additionally, it can prevent the implantation of a fertilized egg by altering the endometrial lining of the uterus.

B. Effectiveness and Reliability

Postinor 2 is most effective when taken as soon as possible after unprotected intercourse. Its effectiveness diminishes the longer the delay in taking the pill:

- **Within 24 hours:** Approximately 95% effective.

- **Within 48 hours:** Approximately 85% effective.

- **Within 72 hours:** Approximately 58% effective.

While highly effective, it is not 100% foolproof, and its efficacy decreases significantly after 72 hours.

C. Usage Instructions

When and How to Take It

Postinor 2 should be taken as soon as possible after unprotected sex, ideally within 72 hours. The sooner it is taken, the more effective it will be. It is available over-the-counter in many countries, making it accessible without a prescription.

Dosage Information

Postinor 2 typically comes in a single-dose pill containing 1.5 mg of levonorgestrel. In some formulations, it is provided as two 0.75 mg tablets, taken 12 hours apart. However, taking both tablets at once is equally effective.

D. Side Effects and Risks

Common Side Effects

- **Nausea and Vomiting:** Some women may experience nausea or vomiting after taking Postinor 2. If vomiting occurs within two hours of taking the pill, another dose may be necessary.

- **Fatigue:** Feeling tired is a common side effect.

- **Dizziness:** Some women may feel lightheaded or dizzy.

- **Breast Tenderness:** Tender or sore breasts can occur.

- **Headache:** Headaches are a possible side effect.

- **Menstrual Changes:** The next period may be earlier, later, heavier, or lighter than usual.

E. Potential Risks and How to Manage Them

- **Ectopic Pregnancy:** While rare, there is a small risk of ectopic pregnancy (a pregnancy that implants outside the uterus). Seek immediate medical attention if experiencing severe abdominal pain.

- **Menstrual Irregularities:** If menstrual changes persist or if the period is more than a week late, a pregnancy test is recommended.

- **Allergic Reactions:** Severe allergic reactions are rare but can occur. Symptoms may include rash, itching, swelling, and difficulty breathing.

Immediate medical attention is required if these occur.

Managing side effects involves supportive care and monitoring for any severe reactions. Over-the-counter medications can help alleviate symptoms like headaches and nausea. Maintaining hydration and rest can also help manage minor side effects. If severe side effects or unusual symptoms occur, it is important to consult a healthcare professional.

By understanding Postinor 2, its usage, and potential side effects, women can make informed decisions about their reproductive health and emergency contraception options.

CHAPTER TWO

POSTINOR 2 IN CONTEXT

2.1 Comparing Emergency Contraceptives

A. Different Types of Emergency Contraceptives

There are several types of emergency contraceptives available, each with its own mechanisms and characteristics. The primary options include:

1. **Levonorgestrel-based Pills (e.g., Postinor 2)**

   o Contains levonorgestrel, a synthetic progestin hormone.

- Most effective when taken within 72 hours of unprotected intercourse.

2. **Ulipristal Acetate (e.g., Ella)**

   - Contains ulipristal acetate, a selective progesterone receptor modulator.

   - Can be taken up to 120 hours (5 days) after unprotected sex.

   - Requires a prescription in many countries.

3. **Copper Intrauterine Device (IUD)**

   - Non-hormonal method, involves inserting a copper IUD into the uterus.

- o Can be used as emergency contraception if inserted within 5 days of unprotected sex.

- o Also provides long-term contraception for up to 10 years.

4. **Combined Oral Contraceptives (Yuzpe Regimen)**

- o Uses higher doses of regular birth control pills containing both estrogen and progestin.

- o Less commonly used due to higher incidence of side effects.

B. Pros and Cons of Each

1. **Levonorgestrel-based Pills**

   - **Pros:** Widely available over-the-counter, effective within a short window, minimal side effects.

   - **Cons:** Decreases in effectiveness after 72 hours, not effective if ovulation has already occurred.

2. **Ulipristal Acetate**

   - **Pros:** Effective up to 5 days after intercourse, slightly more effective than levonorgestrel-based pills.

- o **Cons:** Requires a prescription, potential interactions with hormonal contraceptives.

3. **Copper IUD**

   - o **Pros:** Highly effective, works up to 5 days after intercourse, provides long-term contraception.

   - o **Cons:** Requires insertion by a healthcare provider, may cause discomfort during insertion, more expensive upfront.

4. **Combined Oral Contraceptives**

- o **Pros:** Can be used if other methods are not available, familiar to users of regular birth control pills.

- o **Cons:** Higher risk of side effects such as nausea and vomiting, less effective compared to other methods.

2.2 Myths and Facts

A. Common Misconceptions about Postinor 2

- **Myth:** Postinor 2 causes abortion.

  - o **Fact:** Postinor 2 does not terminate an existing pregnancy. It prevents pregnancy by inhibiting ovulation, fertilization, or implantation.

- **Myth:** Postinor 2 is 100% effective.

  - **Fact:** While highly effective, Postinor 2 is not foolproof. Its effectiveness decreases the longer the delay in taking it after unprotected sex.

- **Myth:** Postinor 2 can be used as a regular contraceptive.

  - **Fact:** Postinor 2 is designed for emergency use only and is not as effective as regular contraceptive methods for ongoing prevention of pregnancy.

- **Myth:** Taking Postinor 2 multiple times is harmful.

  - o **Fact:** There is no evidence that occasional use of Postinor 2 is harmful, but it should not replace regular contraception due to potential for menstrual irregularities.

2.3 Evidence-Based Facts to Dispel Myths

- **Fact:** Postinor 2 is safe for most women and has been extensively studied to ensure its safety and efficacy.

- **Fact:** The World Health Organization (WHO) recognizes levonorgestrel-based emergency contraceptives as a safe and effective method for preventing unintended pregnancy.

- **Fact:** Postinor 2 does not affect future fertility; women can conceive in the future after using it.

2.4 Legal and Ethical Considerations

A. Legal Status Around the World

- **Over-the-Counter Availability:** In many countries, Postinor 2 is available over-the-counter without a prescription, making it easily accessible for women in need of emergency contraception.

- **Prescription Requirements:** In some regions, a prescription is required to obtain Postinor 2, which can limit accessibility, especially in urgent situations.

- **Age Restrictions:** Certain countries have age restrictions for purchasing emergency contraception, requiring younger women to obtain a prescription or parental consent.

B. Ethical Debates and Perspectives

- **Access and Autonomy:** Advocates argue that women should have unrestricted access to emergency contraception to maintain control over their reproductive health and prevent unintended pregnancies.

- **Moral and Religious Views:** Some oppose emergency contraception on moral or religious grounds, believing it interferes with natural reproductive processes. These views can influence policies and access.

- **Public Health Perspective:** Public health officials emphasize the importance of emergency contraception in reducing unintended pregnancies and associated health and social issues. They advocate for wider access and education.

By understanding the various emergency contraceptive options, debunking common myths, and considering the legal and ethical dimensions, readers can gain a comprehensive perspective on Postinor 2 and its role in women's health.

CHAPTER THREE

POSTINOR 2 AND WOMEN'S HEALTH

3.1 Reproductive Health

A. Impact on Menstrual Cycle

Postinor 2 can affect a woman's menstrual cycle in several ways. Most women will experience changes in their next period after taking the pill. These changes might include:

- **Timing:** The next period may come earlier or later than expected.

- **Flow:** The menstrual flow might be heavier or lighter than usual.

- **Duration:** The duration of the period can also be affected, potentially being shorter or longer.

These changes are typically temporary and should normalize by the following cycle. However, if menstrual irregularities persist, it's advisable to consult a healthcare provider.

B. Long-Term Reproductive Health Considerations

Postinor 2 is intended for occasional use and is not meant to replace regular contraceptive methods. Its impact on long-term reproductive health is minimal when used as directed. Key considerations include:

- **Fertility:** There is no evidence to suggest that Postinor 2 affects long-term fertility. Women can conceive in future cycles after using the pill.

- **Frequent Use:** Using Postinor 2 frequently can lead to menstrual irregularities. It is not recommended as a regular contraceptive method due to its lower effectiveness compared to other forms of contraception.

Regular use of more reliable contraception, such as birth control pills, IUDs, or implants, is recommended for ongoing prevention of pregnancy and to maintain stable reproductive health.

3.2 Emotional and Mental Health

A. Emotional Responses and Mental Health Impact

Taking emergency contraception can evoke a range of emotional responses. Common feelings include:

- **Relief:** Many women feel relieved knowing they have taken steps to prevent an unintended pregnancy.

- **Anxiety:** There can be anxiety about the effectiveness of the pill and potential side effects.

- **Guilt or Shame:** Some women may experience feelings of guilt or shame due to societal or personal beliefs about contraception.

B. Coping Strategies and Support Resources

Managing emotional and mental health is crucial after using emergency contraception. Strategies include:

- **Education:** Understanding how Postinor 2 works and its safety can alleviate anxiety.

- **Support Networks:** Talking to trusted friends, family members, or partners can provide emotional support.

- **Professional Counseling:** Seeking help from a counselor or therapist can be beneficial, especially if feelings of guilt, shame, or anxiety are overwhelming.

- **Support Groups:** Joining support groups, either in person or online, can connect women with others who have had similar experiences.

3.3 Postinor 2 and Adolescents

A. Special Considerations for Teenage Users

Adolescents may face unique challenges when it comes to using emergency contraception like Postinor 2:

- **Access:** Teens may have limited access due to age restrictions or lack of information about where to obtain the pill.

- **Education:** There may be gaps in knowledge about how to use emergency contraception correctly and its potential effects.

- **Stigma:** Adolescents might feel stigmatized or judged for seeking out or using emergency contraception.

B. Education and Communication Strategies for Parents and Guardians

Parents and guardians play a crucial role in educating and supporting adolescents regarding emergency contraception:

- **Open Communication:** Encourage open, honest discussions about sexual health and contraception without judgment or criticism. Create a safe space for teens to ask questions and express their concerns.

- **Accurate Information:** Provide accurate, age-appropriate information about Postinor 2, including how it works, when to use it, and potential side effects.

- **Access to Resources:** Ensure that adolescents know where and how to access emergency contraception. This might include providing information about local pharmacies, clinics, and hotlines.

- **Encouraging Responsibility:** Emphasize the importance of using regular contraception to prevent unintended pregnancies and reduce the need for emergency contraception.

By understanding the impacts of Postinor 2

on menstrual cycles, long-term reproductive

health, emotional well-being, and the specific

considerations for adolescent users, readers

can better navigate the use of emergency

contraception and support those who may

need it. Providing education and fostering

open communication are essential steps in

promoting informed and responsible use of

Postinor 2.

CHAPTER FOUR

ACCESS AND ADVOCACY

4.1 Accessibility and Availability

A. How to Obtain Postinor 2

Postinor 2 is widely available in many countries and can often be obtained through the following means:

1. **Over-the-Counter (OTC) Sales:** In many countries, Postinor 2 is available without a prescription at pharmacies. This allows for quick and easy access.

2. **Prescription:** In some regions, a prescription from a healthcare provider is required. This may necessitate a visit to a clinic or doctor.

3. **Online Pharmacies:** Some reputable online pharmacies offer Postinor 2 for purchase. It's important to ensure the online source is legitimate to avoid counterfeit medications.

4. **Health Clinics and Family Planning Centers:** Many health clinics and family planning centers provide emergency contraception. Some may offer it for free or at a reduced cost.

4.2 Barriers to Access and How to Overcome Them

Despite its availability, there are several barriers that can impede access to Postinor 2:

1. **Legal and Regulatory Restrictions:** In some countries, stringent regulations limit the availability of emergency contraception. Advocacy for policy changes can help improve access.

2. **Cost:** The price of Postinor 2 can be prohibitive for some individuals. Subsidized programs and insurance coverage can help mitigate this barrier.

3. **Lack of Awareness:** Many people may not be aware of the availability or proper use of Postinor 2. Public health campaigns and education can address this issue.

4. **Stigma and Judgment:** Cultural and societal stigma around emergency contraception can discourage individuals from seeking it. Creating a supportive environment and promoting positive attitudes toward reproductive health can help overcome this barrier.

5. **Geographical Barriers:** In remote or rural areas, access to pharmacies and healthcare facilities may be limited.

Mobile health clinics and telemedicine can provide alternatives for these populations.

4.3 Advocacy and Support

A. Organizations Supporting Women's Access to Contraception

Numerous organizations work to improve access to contraception and support women's reproductive rights. Some key organizations include:

1. **Planned Parenthood:** Provides comprehensive reproductive health services and advocates for women's health and rights.

2. **Marie Stopes International:** Offers contraception and safe abortion services globally, with a focus on underserved populations.

3. **International Planned Parenthood Federation (IPPF):** Advocates for sexual and reproductive health and rights worldwide.

4. **The Guttmacher Institute:** Conducts research and policy analysis on reproductive health issues.

5. **UNFPA (United Nations Population Fund):** Works to ensure universal access to reproductive

health services, including family planning.

B. How to Advocate for Better Reproductive Health Policies

Advocacy for better reproductive health policies involves several strategies:

1. **Educate and Raise Awareness:** Inform the public and policymakers about the importance of accessible contraception and the benefits it provides for women's health and societal well-being.

2. **Engage with Policymakers:** Meet with local, regional, and national policymakers to discuss the need for

improved access to emergency contraception and other reproductive health services.

3. **Support Reproductive Health Legislation:** Advocate for the passage of laws that protect and expand access to reproductive health services. This can include writing letters, signing petitions, and participating in public hearings.

4. **Collaborate with Advocacy Groups:** Partner with organizations that focus on reproductive rights to strengthen advocacy efforts. Joint campaigns and coalition-building can

amplify the impact of advocacy initiatives.

5. **Utilize Media and Social Platforms:** Use traditional and social media to spread awareness and advocate for policy changes. Writing op-eds, sharing stories, and engaging in online discussions can help mobilize public support.

6. **Promote Comprehensive Sex Education:** Advocate for sex education programs that include information about emergency contraception and reproductive health. Education is a critical component of empowering

individuals to make informed decisions.

By understanding how to obtain Postinor 2, recognizing and addressing barriers to access, and actively engaging in advocacy and support efforts, readers can contribute to improving reproductive health access and policies. Ensuring that emergency contraception is readily available and that women have the necessary support and information is vital for promoting reproductive rights and health.

CHAPTER FIVE

FREQUENTLY ASKED QUESTIONS

5.1 Common Questions

A. Addressing Frequently Asked Questions About Postinor 2

1. **What is Postinor 2?**

   o Postinor 2 is an emergency contraceptive pill containing levonorgestrel, used to prevent pregnancy after unprotected sex or contraceptive failure.

2. **How does Postinor 2 work?**

- Postinor 2 primarily works by preventing or delaying ovulation. It may also prevent fertilization or implantation of a fertilized egg by altering the uterine lining.

3. **When should I take Postinor 2?**

   - For maximum effectiveness, take Postinor 2 as soon as possible after unprotected sex, ideally within 72 hours. The sooner it is taken, the more effective it will be.

4. **How effective is Postinor 2?**

   - Postinor 2 is most effective when taken within 24 hours of unprotected sex, with an effectiveness of approximately 95%. Its effectiveness decreases to around 85% if taken within 48 hours and about 58% if taken within 72 hours.

5. **Can I use Postinor 2 as regular contraception?**

   o No, Postinor 2 is designed for emergency use only and is not as effective as regular contraceptive methods for ongoing prevention of pregnancy.

6. **What are the side effects of Postinor 2?**

- Common side effects include nausea, fatigue, dizziness, breast tenderness, headache, and changes in menstrual bleeding. These effects are usually temporary.

7. **Does Postinor 2 affect my future fertility?**

- No, Postinor 2 does not have long-term effects on fertility. It is safe to use, and you can still conceive in the future.

8. **What should I do if I vomit after taking Postinor 2?**

- o If you vomit within two hours of taking Postinor 2, you may need to take another dose. Consult a healthcare provider for guidance.

9. **Can I take Postinor 2 if I'm already using regular contraception?**

- o Yes, if you experience contraceptive failure (e.g., a condom breaks), you can take Postinor 2 as an emergency measure.

10. **What should I do if my period is late after taking Postinor 2?**

- o A delay in your period can occur after taking Postinor 2.

If your period is more than a week late, it is advisable to take a pregnancy test and consult a healthcare provider.

5.2 Expert Answers

A. Providing Clear and Accurate Answers Based on Medical Expertise

1. **Is Postinor 2 safe for all women to use?**

   o Yes, Postinor 2 is generally safe for most women. However, it is always best to consult a healthcare provider if you have any underlying

medical   conditions   or
concerns.

2. **Can Postinor 2 be used multiple
    times in one menstrual cycle?**

    o   While it is safe to use Postinor

        2 more than once in a cycle if

        necessary, it should not be

        used   as   a   regular

        contraceptive   method.

        Frequent use can lead to

        menstrual irregularities.

3. **What is the difference between
    Postinor 2 and regular birth
    control pills?**

    o   Postinor 2 is an emergency

        contraceptive   meant   for

occasional use, containing a higher dose of levonorgestrel compared to regular birth control pills. Regular birth control pills are taken daily and are more effective for ongoing contraception.

4. **How does Postinor 2 compare to other emergency contraceptives like Ella or the Copper IUD?**

   o Postinor 2 (levonorgestrel) is effective within 72 hours of unprotected sex. Ella (ulipristal acetate) can be used up to 120 hours after. The Copper IUD is the most effective emergency contraceptive and can be used up to 5 days after unprotected sex, also providing long-term contraception.

5. **Can Postinor 2 cause an abortion?**

    o   No, Postinor 2 does not cause an abortion. It prevents pregnancy by inhibiting ovulation, fertilization, or implantation. It is ineffective if implantation has already occurred.

6. **Are there any medical conditions that would prevent someone from using Postinor 2?**

- o   Most women can safely use Postinor 2. However, those with severe liver disease, certain rare hereditary problems of galactose intolerance, or glucose-galactose malabsorption should consult a healthcare provider before use.

7. **Is Postinor 2 effective against sexually transmitted infections (STIs)?**

    - o   No, Postinor 2 does not protect against STIs. Using condoms is recommended to reduce the risk of STIs.

8. **What should I do if I suspect I am pregnant after taking Postinor 2?**

   o If you suspect pregnancy after taking Postinor 2 (e.g., your period is more than a week late), take a pregnancy test and consult a healthcare provider for further advice and care.

9. **Can adolescents use Postinor 2?**

   o Yes, Postinor 2 is safe for use by adolescents. However, they should be educated on proper usage and the importance of regular contraception.

10. **How should Postinor 2 be stored?**

- o Store Postinor 2 at room temperature, away from direct sunlight and moisture. Keep it out of reach of children.

By addressing these common questions with expert answers, readers can gain a comprehensive understanding of Postinor 2, its use, and its effects. Clear and accurate information is crucial for making informed decisions about emergency contraception and reproductive health.

CHAPTER SIX

ADDITIONAL RESOURCES

6.1 Educational Materials

Books, Articles, and Websites for Further Reading

1. **Books:**

   o "Taking Charge of Your Fertility" by Toni Weschler: A comprehensive guide to understanding your reproductive health.

   o "Emergency Contraception: The Story of a Global Reproductive Health

Technology" by A. Rahman and I. Haider: An in-depth look at the history and impact of emergency contraception.

- o "Our Bodies, Ourselves" by the Boston Women's Health Book Collective: A classic resource on women's health and reproductive rights.

2. **Articles:**

- o "Emergency Contraception: A Last Chance to Prevent Unintended Pregnancy" by the American College of Obstetricians and Gynecologists: An overview of emergency contraception options and their use.

- o "The Impact of Emergency Contraception on Women's Health" by the Guttmacher Institute: Research on the benefits and challenges of emergency contraception access.

3. **Websites:**

- o **Planned Parenthood (www.plannedparenthood.org):** Provides information on emergency contraception, reproductive health, and available services.

- o **The American College of Obstetricians and Gynecologists (www.acog.org):** Offers clinical guidance and patient education on a wide range of reproductive health topics.

- o **Bedsider (www.bedsider.org):** A resource for birth control and emergency contraception information, including methods, effectiveness, and side effects.

6.2 Support Services

**Hotlines, Support Groups, and
Counseling Services**

1. **Hotlines:**

    o   **Planned   Parenthood
        Hotline:** 1-800-230-PLAN
        (7526): Provides information
        and support on reproductive
        health and contraception.

    o   **National   Sexual   Assault
        Hotline:** 1-800-656-HOPE
        (4673): Offers confidential
        support for sexual assault
        survivors,   including
        information on emergency
        contraception.

2. **Support Groups:**

   o **Sexual Health and Reproductive Rights Groups:** Many local and online communities offer support and education on reproductive health and contraception.

   o **Online Forums:** Websites like Reddit and specialized health forums provide platforms for sharing experiences and advice.

3. **Counseling Services:**

   o **Family Planning Clinics:** Offer counseling on

contraception, sexual health, and pregnancy options.

- o **Mental Health Counselors:** Specialized in reproductive health and emotional well-being, they can help manage any emotional responses to using emergency contraception.

Healthcare Providers

How to Find a Healthcare Provider for Reproductive Health

1. **Local Health Clinics and Hospitals:**

- o Visit local health clinics and hospitals for referrals to gynecologists, obstetricians, and reproductive health specialists.

2. **Planned Parenthood Centers:**

   - o Use the Planned Parenthood website to find local centers offering reproductive health services, including emergency contraception and counseling.

3. **Primary Care Providers:**

   - o Consult your primary care provider for referrals to

specialists in reproductive health.

4. **Online Directories:**

o Use online directories like Zocdoc, Healthgrades, or the American College of Obstetricians and Gynecologists' "Find an Ob-Gyn" tool to locate qualified healthcare providers in your area.

6.3 Conclusion

A. Summary of Key Points

- Postinor 2 is an effective emergency contraceptive intended for occasional use.

- Understanding how Postinor 2 works, its side effects, and proper usage is crucial for making informed decisions.

- Access to Postinor 2 varies globally, with barriers including cost, legal restrictions, and lack of awareness.

- Emotional and mental health considerations are important when using emergency contraception, with various support resources available.

- Advocacy and education play key roles in improving access to emergency contraception and reproductive health services.

B. Final Thoughts

Emergency contraception like Postinor 2 empowers women to take control of their reproductive health. While it is a valuable option for preventing unintended pregnancy, regular contraception methods should be used for ongoing prevention. Access to accurate information, support services, and healthcare providers is essential for making informed decisions.

Encouragement and Support for Readers

Taking charge of your reproductive health is a vital step towards empowerment and well-being. It's normal to have questions and concerns, and there are many resources and supportive communities available to help. Educate yourself, seek support when needed, and make informed choices that best suit your needs and lifestyle.

C. Call to Action

How Readers Can Take Charge of Their Reproductive Health

1. **Educate Yourself:** Stay informed about reproductive health, contraception options, and your rights.

2. **Seek Support:** Utilize available resources, such as hotlines, counseling services, and support groups, to navigate your reproductive health journey.

3. **Advocate:** Support and advocate for better access to contraception and reproductive health services in your community and beyond.

4. **Communicate:** Have open and honest conversations with partners, healthcare providers, and loved ones about your reproductive health needs and concerns.

5. **Take Action:** Be proactive in managing your reproductive health

by scheduling regular check-ups, using contraception effectively, and knowing where to access emergency contraception if needed.

By taking these steps, you can ensure that you are well-prepared to handle your reproductive health with confidence and support.

www.ingramcontent.com/pod-product-compliance
Lightning Source LLC
Chambersburg PA
CBHW051654250726

48653CB00007B/2665